1. Prevalence of Diabetes mellitus in pregnancy is:
A) 5.4%
B) 6%
C) 8%
D) 10%
E) 12%

Ans: A)

2. Most common type of diabetes mellitus in pregnancy is:
A) Gestational diabetes mellitus
B) Type II Diabetes mellitus
C) Type I Diabetes mellitus
D) All in equal proportion
E) juvenile onset diabetes mellitus.

Ans: A)

Approximately 87.5% have gestational diabetes (which may or may not resolve after pregnancy), 7.5% have type1 diabetes and the remaining 5% have type2 diabetes. The prevalence of type1 diabetes, and especially type2 diabetes, has increased in recent years

3. Condition related to type I DM are:
A) Hashimoto`s thyroiditis,
B) Graves' disease,
C) Addison`s disease,
D) Vitiligo
E) All of the above

Ans: E)

Hashimoto`s thyroiditis, Graves' disease, Addison`s disease, vitiligo, celiac sprue, autoimmune hepatitis, myasthenia gravis, and pernicious anaemia associated with it.

HLA on chromosome 6 is responsible, but vertical transmission is low and concordance rate for twin is less than 50%.

4. Offer women with following risk factors for gestational diabetes, a 75g 2-hour OGTT at 24–28weeks except:

A) BMI above 30kg/m^2

B) Previous macrosomic baby weighing 4.5kg or above

C) Previous gestational diabetes

D) Family history of diabetes (first-degree relative with diabetes)

E) Minority ethnic family origin with a high prevalence of diabetes

Ans: C

Offer women who have had gestational diabetes in a previous pregnancy: early self-monitoring of blood glucose OR a 75g 2-hour OGTT as soon as possible after booking (whether in the first or second trimester), and a further 75g 2-hour OGTT at 24–28weeks if the results of the first OGTT are normal.)

(Offer women with any of the other risk factors for gestational diabetes a 75g 2-hour OGTT at 24–28weeks.)

5. Impact of overt diabetes on pregnancy is:

A) Spontaneous miscarriage

B) Preterm labor

C) Malformations

D) FGR

E) All of the above

Ans: E

Foetal effects:

a) Spontaneous abortions: HbA1c >7% or plasma glucose >120mg/dl associated with three fold increase in risk of spontaneous abortion.

b) Preterm delivery: 26% (6.8% in normal population) rate of preterm delivery in overt diabetic population.

c) Malformation: in type 1 DM incidence is double (5%). Half are cardiovascular anomalies (there is fourfold increase in cardiac anomalies as compared to non-cardiac anomalies). Incidence of various anomalies is: Cardiovascular(52%), Musculoskeletal (12%), Urogenital (9%), CNS (4%),

Gastrointestinal (2%), Chromosomal (3%), Other (10%), Multi-organ(8%). Although caudal regression is rare malformation it is frequently associated with maternal diabetes. The frequency of major congenital malformation in new-born with pregestational diabetes according to HBA1c in first visit:

<6% HBA1c   : 2.8%
6-6.9HBA1c%   : 5%
7-7.9%HBA1c   : 11.7%
8%HBA1c >=   : 15.8%

Possible explanation is: Hyperglycaemia produces toxic radical and initiate programmed cell death. Also it is observed that hyperglycaemia oxidative stress inhibit migration of cardiac neural-crest cell in embryo of diabetic mice.

d) Altered foetal growth :

Diminished foetal growth: more typical of pre-gestational diabetes mellitus. Results from congenital malformation or from substrate deprivation due to advanced vascular disease.

Macrosomia: particularly in second half of gestation maternal hyperglycaemia prompts foetal hyperinsulinemia which cause macrosomia. Except brain most of part affected. There is deposition of fat on shoulder, trunk which may cause shoulder dystocia. Incidence of macrosomia rises with increase in maternal plasma glucose level more than 130mg/dl. Incidence of macrosomia in type 1, type 2 and gestational diabetes mellitus is 35%,28%,24% respectively.

e) Unexplained foetal demise:

Three times more in type 1 DM as compared to general obstetrical population. Stillbirths generally occur after 35 weeks before labour and babies are typically large for gestational age. The cause is unexplained (because common causes like obvious placental insufficiency, abruption, foetal growth restriction, or oligohydramnios are not identified). These unexplained stillbirth commonly (2/3rd of cases) associated with poor glycaemic control. This may be due to hyperglycaemia mediated chronic aberrations in oxygen and foetal metabolic transport. This is supported by study conducted by Salvesen which show mean umbilical vein ph is less in diabetic pregnancy. Also there is 7 fold increase in unexplained stillbirth in pregnancy associated with both diabetes and PIH as compared to 3 fold increase in diabetes alone.

f) Hydramnios (AFI >24CM): women with elevated HbA1c and uncontrolled sugar level found to have more incidence of polyhydramnios in third trimester.

g) Neonatal effect: increased neonatal morbidity due to preterm birth and early induction to avoid unexplained stillbirth.

h) Respiratory distress syndrome: historically, new-borns of diabetic mothers were thought to be at increased risk for respiratory distress from delayed lung maturation. But recent study by Bental and colleague fails to demonstrate this concept. Gestational age is more important factor.

i) Hypoglycaemia: because of hyperplasia of beta islet cells induced by chronic maternal hyperglycaemia, new-born of diabetic mother experience rapid drop in plasma glucose concentration. Low glycaemia defined by plasma glucose level below 45mg/dl. Prompt recognition and monitoring decrease incidence of hypoglycaemia.

j) Hypocalcaemia: it is defined as serum level less than 8 mg/dl in term neonates. Every third patient in uncontrolled diabetes mellitus developed hypocalcaemia as compared to controlled diabetes where incidence is 18%.

k) Hyperbilirubinemia and polycythaemia: polycythaemia is thought to be due to chronic hypoxia induced by hyperglycaemia. Hyperglycaemia in mother consumed more oxygen depriving foetus of oxygen. This hypoxia induces increase erythropoietin. Increase erythropoietin along with increase insulin cause polycythaemia. Polycythaemia cause increase bilirubin. 40 % of neonate show haematocrits of 65-70% volume.

l) Cardiomyopathy: primarily affect interventricular septum followed by right ventricle. In severe cases cardiomyopathy leads to obstructive cardiac failure.

Structural changes precede cardiac failure. Most of affected new born asymptomatic at birth and hypertrophy resolved in months after birth because of relief from maternal hyperglycaemia. Conversely foetal cardiomyopathy may progress to adult cardiomyopathy.

m) Long term cognitive development: Despite of rigorous antepartum management intelligence quotient (by 1 to 2 points) and memory is less in babies of mother with overt diabetes in pregnancy. Also incidence of autism is more.

n) Inheritance of diabetes: risk of developing type 1 if either parent affected is 3 or 4 %. If both parent have type 2 DM then incidence of inheritance is 40%. It is observed that breast feeding increase incidence of developing type 1 DM and decrease incidence of type 2 DM.

6. Before conception women with diabetes should maintain pre-prandial glucose level between:

A) 70 to 100 mg/dl
B) 100 to 120 mg/dl
C) 120 to 140mg/dl
D) 140 to 180mg/dl
E) 180 to 200 mg/dl

Ans: A

7. Women with type I and II DM in pregnancy should offered induction of labor :

A) Before 37 weeks
B) 37 to 38 + 6 weeks
C) 38 to 39+6 weeks
D) After 40 weeks
E) Do not offer induction of labor

Ans: B

8. On screening test Diagnosis of gestational diabetes mellitus is made when:

37+0 weeks to 38+6 weeks	Offer induction of labour, or caesarean section if indicated, to women with type1 or type2 diabetes; otherwise await spontaneous labour.
38weeks	Offer tests of foetal wellbeing.
39weeks	Offer tests of foetal wellbeing. Advise women with uncomplicated gestational diabetes to give birth no later than 40+6 weeks.

A) A fasting plasma glucose level of 5.6mmol/litre (100mg/dl) or above

B) A 2-hour plasma glucose level of 7.8mmol/litre (140mg/dl) or above

C) A fasting plasma glucose level of 7.8mmol/litre (100mg/dl) or above

D) Either A or B

E) Both A and B should present

Ans: D

Diagnose gestational diabetes if the woman has either:

-A fasting plasma glucose level of 5.6mmol/litre (100mg/dl) or above

-A 2-hour plasma glucose level of 7.8mmol/litre (140mg/dl) or above

9. For every 1 Kg/m² increase in BMI prevalence of GDM increase by

  A) 1%

  B) 2%

  C) 10%

  D) 20%

  E) 30%

  Ans: A

  10. Women with type I DM in pregnancy should test for following daily:
  A) Fasting blood glucose
  B) Pre-meal blood glucose
  C) 1 hour post meal glucose
  D) Bed time blood glucose

E) All of the above

Ans: E

Monitoring blood glucose:

1. Advise pregnant women with type1 diabetes to test their fasting, pre-meal, 1-hour post-meal and bedtime blood glucose levels daily during pregnancy.

2. Advise pregnant women with type2 diabetes or gestational diabetes who are on a multiple daily insulin injection regimen to test their fasting, pre-meal, 1-hour post-meal and bedtime blood glucose levels daily during pregnancy.

3. Advise pregnant women with type2 diabetes or gestational diabetes to test their fasting and 1-hour post-meal blood glucose levels daily during pregnancy if they are:

-on diet and exercise therapy

-taking oral therapy (with or without diet and exercise therapy) or single-dose intermediate-acting or long-acting insulin

11. Immediate treatment with insulin should be started when fasting blood glucose become:

A) 7.0mmol/litre and above

B) 6.0mmol/litre and above

c) *between 6.0 and 6.9mmol/litre(108 to 124mg/dl) if there are complications such as macrosomia or hydramnios.*

D) A and c

E) A and B

Ans: D

12. Advise pregnant women with any form of diabetes to maintain their capillary plasma glucose below the following target levels, if these are achievable without causing problematic hypoglycaemia
A) Fasting: 5.3mmol/litre (96mg/dl)
B) Fasting: 7.8mmol/litre (96mg/dl)
C) A,D and E

D) 1hour after meals: 7.8mmol/litre (140mg/dl)

E) 2hours after meals: 6.4mmol/litre (116mg/dl)

Ans: C

13. Consider Glibenclamide for women with gestational diabetes:

A) in whom blood glucose targets are not achieved with metformin but who decline insulin therapy

B) who cannot tolerate metformin.

C) In all women

D) A and B

E) Women not controlled on medical nutritional therapy

Ans: D

14. The American College of Obstetricians and Gynecologists (2013) has suggested that caesarean delivery should be considered in women with gestational diabetes whose foetuses have a sonographically estimated weight

A) ≥ 4500 g.

B) 5000 g
C) 4000g
D) 3500g
E) 5000g

Ans: A

15. Drug not to be used for tocolysis in women with diabetes in pregnancy is:
A) Calcium channel blocker
B) Magnesium sulphate
C) Atosiban
D) Beta mimetic
E) Nitroglycerine
    Ans: D

16. capillary plasma glucose should be monitor every ___hour in labor
A) 1
B) 2
C) 3
D) 4
E) 5
    Ans: A

17. capillary plasma glucose in labor should be maintain between:

A) 4 mmol/litre (72mg/dl) to
   7mmol/litre (126mg/dl)
B) 7 to 10 mmol
C) 10 to 14 mmol
D) Less than 14 mmol
E) None of the above

Ans: A

In a gestational diabetic the requirement of insulin is likely to fall precipitously and no insulin may be required immediately after expulsion of placenta.

Monitor capillary plasma glucose every hour during labour and birth in women with diabetes, and ensure that it is maintained between 4 mmol/litre (72mg/dl) to 7mmol/litre (126mg/dl).

Intravenous dextrose and insulin infusion should be considered for women with type1 diabetes from the onset of established labour.

18. capillary plasma glucose should be monitor every ___hour in general anaesthesia:

A) ½
B) 1
C) 2
D) 3
E) 4

Ans: A

19. Which of the following is not true about newborn care of diabetes mother:

A) Early clamping of the cord, i.e. within 20 seconds of delivery, to avoid erythrocytosis.

B) Late clamping of the cord, i.e. after 20 seconds of delivery, to avoid erythrocytosis.

C) Perform a preliminary physical examination to detect major congenital malformations

D) Monitor heart and respiratory rates, colour, and motor behaviour for at least the first 24 hours after birth

E) Carry out blood glucose testing routinely in babies of women with diabetes at 2–4hours after birth

Ans: B

As soon as the infant is born, the following actions are mandatory:

-Early clamping of the cord, i.e. within 20 seconds of delivery, to avoid erythrocytosis.

-Evaluate vital signs; Apgar scores at 1 and 5 minutes;

-Clear oropharynx and nose of mucus; later empty the stomach - be aware that stimulation of the pharynx with the catheter may lead to reflex bradycardia and apnoea;

-Avoid heat loss, keep neonate warm, and transfer to incubator pre-warmed to 34^0C;

-Perform a preliminary physical examination to detect major congenital malformations;

-Monitor heart and respiratory rates, colour, and motor behaviour for at least the first 24 hours after birth;

-Women with diabetes should feed their babies as soon as possible after birth (within 30minutes) and then at frequent intervals (every 2–3hours) until feeding maintains pre-feed capillary plasma glucose levels at a minimum of 2.0mmol/litre(36mg/dl). Aim at full caloric intake (125 kcal/kg/24 hours) at 5 days, divided into six to eight feeds a day.

-Carry out blood glucose testing routinely in babies of women with diabetes at 2–4hours after birth. Carry out blood tests for polycythaemia, hyperbilirubinaemia, hypocalcaemia and hypomagnesaemia for babies with clinical signs. Perform an echocardiogram for babies of women with diabetes if they show clinical signs associated with congenital heart disease or cardiomyopathy, including heart murmur. The timing of the examination will depend on the clinical circumstances.

-If capillary plasma glucose values are below 2.0mmol/litre on 2consecutive readings despite maximal support for feeding, if there are abnormal clinical signs or if the baby will not feed orally effectively, use additional measures such as tube feeding or intravenous dextrose. Only implement additional measures if one or more of these criteria are met.

20. For women who were diagnosed with gestational diabetes and whose blood glucose levels returned to normal after the birth

A) Offer lifestyle advice (including weight control, diet and exercise).

B) Offer a fasting plasma glucose test 6–13weeks after the birth to exclude diabetes (for practical reasons this might take place at the 6-week postnatal check).

C) If a fasting plasma glucose test has not been performed by 13weeks, offer a fasting plasma glucose test, or an HbA1c test if a fasting plasma glucose test is not possible, after 13weeks.

D) Do not routinely offer a 75g 2-hour OGTT.

E) Offer an annual HbA1c test to women who were diagnosed with gestational diabetes who have a negative postnatal test for diabetes.

F) All of the above

Ans: F

20. Which of the following is wrong about post partum *advise of women with a fasting plasma glucose level below 6.0mmol/litre (108mg/dl)* :
    A) they have a low probability of having diabetes at present
    B) they should continue to follow the lifestyle advice (including weight control, diet and exercise) given after the birth
    C) they will need an annual test to check that their blood glucose levels are normal.
    D) they have a moderate risk of developing type2 diabetes, and offer them advice and guidance in line with the NICE guideline.
    E) they do not need an annual test to check that their blood glucose levels are normal

    Ans: E

21. Which of the following is CORRECT about post partum

Advice the women with a fasting plasma glucose level between 6.0 and 6.9mmol/litre (108 to 124mg/dl)

A) they have a low probability of having diabetes at present

B) they should continue to follow the lifestyle advice (including weight control, diet and exercise) given after the birth

C) they will need an annual test to check that their blood glucose levels are normal.

D) they have a moderate risk of developing type2 diabetes, and offer them advice and guidance in line with the NICE guideline.

E) they are at high risk of developing type2 diabetes, and offer them advice, guidance and interventions in line with the NICE guideline on preventing type 2 diabetes

Ans: E

Advice the women with fasting plasma glucose level of 7.0mmol/litre or above (126mg/dl): that they are likely to have type2 diabetes, and offer them a diagnostic test to confirm diabetes.

22. Which of the following is wrong about post partum *advise of women an HbA1c level below 39mmol/l (5.7%)* :

A) they have a low probability of having diabetes at present

B) they should continue to follow the lifestyle advice (including weight control, diet and exercise) given after the birth

C) they will need an annual test to check that their blood glucose levels are normal.

D) they have a moderate risk of developing type2 diabetes, and offer them advice and guidance in line with the NICE guideline.

E) they do not need an annual test to check that their blood glucose levels are normal

Ans: E

23. Which of the following is CORRECT about post partum *Advice the women with an HbA1c level between 39 and 47mmol/l (5.7% and 6.4%)*

A) they have a low probability of having diabetes at present

B) they should continue to follow the lifestyle advice (including weight control, diet and exercise) given after the birth

C) they will need an annual test to check that their blood glucose levels are normal.

D) they have a moderate risk of developing type2 diabetes, and offer them advice and guidance in line with the NICE guideline.

E) they are at high risk of developing type2 diabetes, and offer them advice, guidance and interventions in line with the NICE guideline on preventing type 2 diabetes

Ans: E

Advise women with an HbA1c level of 48mmol/l (6.5%) or above that: they have type2 diabetes and refer them for further care.

Women with pre-existing type2 diabetes who are breastfeeding can resume or continue to take metformin [4] and glibenclamide [7] immediately after birth, but should avoid other oral blood glucose-lowering agents while breastfeeding.

www.ingramcontent.com/pod-product-compliance
Lightning Source LLC
Chambersburg PA
CBHW070342190526
45169CB00005B/2003